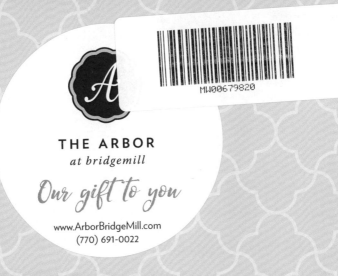

The Journey to Senior Living

A Step-by-Step Guide for Seniors

Printed in the United States of America
First Printing, 2018
ISBN 978-0-692-16053-4

3715 Northside Parkway
Building 300, Suite 110
Atlanta, GA 30327
(404) 237-4026
(404) 237-1719 (Fax)

www.ArborCompany.com

CONTENTS

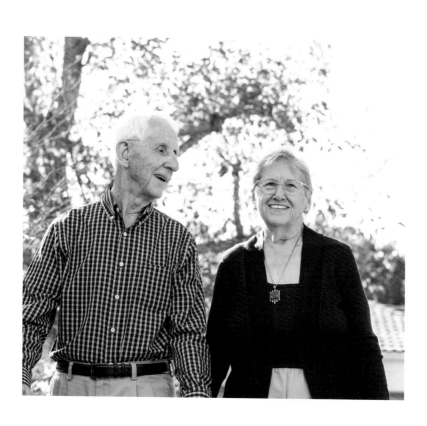

Introduction

Are you contemplating a move to a senior living community? Understandably, you may feel anxious about such a big change. Leaving decades-long homes for someplace new isn't easy. The negative image of nursing homes can be difficult to get past. And like many people, you may think moving to a senior community is surrendering to your age.

Yet, senior living communities can also represent a new adventure. Seniors who have worked hard their whole lives may not want to worry about yard work or property taxes or home maintenance anymore. These same people want to make the most of their retirement, and with luxury and simplicity to fully enjoy friends, family and the joys of daily life, quality senior living emphasizes just that—quality living.

If you are ready for the next chapter of life, senior living—whether it's independent living or assisted living—offers a tremendous opportunity. But the move isn't as simple as a couple phone calls and a quick transition. The journey to senior living requires research, planning and patience. This comprehensive guide offers information and advice to help you find the perfect senior living community and make the transition to your new adventure.

WHY YOU SHOULD TRUST US

The Arbor Company operates more than 30 senior living communities across the nation, and for more than three decades, we have focused on providing quality care to seniors who have a variety of abilities and challenges. While we have won awards for some of our cutting-edge programs, we are more honored when our residents and family members say that moving into an Arbor community was one of the best decisions they ever made. Our local teams work with seniors and their families every day. We know the best parts of senior living, as well as the hard parts. We've taken families through discussions about choosing senior care communities, and we've watched tentative seniors adapt and grow to love their new homes. We can help you through this transition.

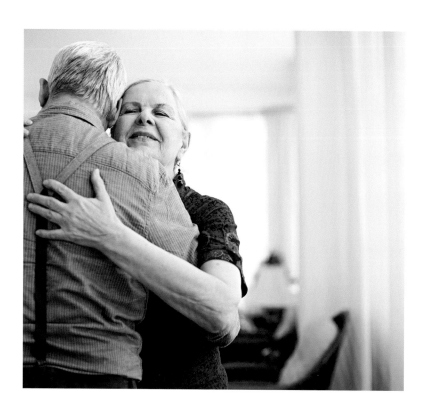

1 | *Is Senior Living Right for You?*

INDEPENDENT LIVING VS. ASSISTED LIVING

The dizzying array of senior living options can be overwhelming. For seniors in reasonably good health, the distinction between assisted and independent living can be especially puzzling. Both options emphasize independence, active living and a sense of community. In both assisted and independent living, seniors typically have their own apartments or condos. Yet, there are some key distinctions between the two models of senior living. Here's what you need to know—and how to choose:

Daily Amenities and Services

Assisted living communities are structured around providing seniors support when and where they need it. Most seniors live in an apartment in close proximity to other community members. Help is often available 24/7 with the simple push of a button, and seniors can get assistance with basic life tasks, including:

- Three meals daily
- Assistance with medications
- Bathing and grooming
- Making and keeping doctor appointments
- Housekeeping and laundry

Assisted living exists on a continuum. Some communities offer more extensive care than others; many provide a range of services that change with a senior's needs and health.

Independent living does not provide medical care or nursing support. Instead, the focus is on convenience and an active life. For example, seniors might be able to order meals or eat at an on-campus cafe, but they are unlikely to get help making nutritional meals or remembering medication unless they hire that extra assistance through a home health agency.

Medical and Supportive Care

Assisted living is a good alternative for people who are no longer able to live alone but do not need intensive nursing care. Independent living preserves a senior's independence, but does not provide access to medical or nursing care unless a home health agency is hired.

Independent living can offer some peace of mind to people who no longer feel comfortable living alone. People with medical conditions that do not undermine the basic activities of daily living may thrive in this environment, but when people are no longer able to tend to their basic needs, make good decisions on their own or function without the help of loved ones, assisted living offers medical support.

Access to and Contact with Staff

In an independent living community, seniors might not have regular contact with the staff unless they sign up for a meal or other service. In these communities, a senior's interaction with staff is largely dependent on the resident's preferences. Someone who eats every meal in the community center might frequently see the staff, but someone who prefers a quieter existence might forget the community even has staff.

In assisted living, staff members monitor and check in on residents. Although staff don't diagnose medical conditions, the team will stay in touch with residents to ensure they are

*"You don't need to be severely ill to decide
assisted living is the better option."*

———

thriving. If a senior appears to need more help,
staff members may drop by more frequently or
talk to the resident's family. A primary benefit of
assisted living is that it offers families peace of
mind knowing that someone is looking out for
their loved ones.

Price

Independent senior living communities are
a living preference—not a form of senior care.
Assisted living, by contrast, greatly expands
upon the level of care a senior would expect at
home. Because of these more extensive services,
assisted living tends to be more costly than
independent living. Assisted living is also more
likely to be covered by long-term care insurance,
employee benefits programs and Medicaid.

Continuum of Care

Seniors residing in assisted living communities
need some degree of support. That may be

something as simple as regular check-ins with a staff member or more extensive support such as help with bathing and grooming.

In many cases, seniors who choose assisted living communities suffer from degenerative health conditions such as Parkinson's, dementia or cancer. They may eventually need more extensive care, so many assisted living communities offer options to transition to nursing or dementia care. In some cases, a senior may be able to continue living in the same place as his or her needs change.

Some independent living communities are associated with assisted living and similar options, but many seniors in independent living communities will continue to lead long and healthy lives without the need for additional care. Therefore, it's less common for independent living providers to offer an extensive continuum of care.

Which Is Right for You?

You don't have to be in perfect health to choose independent living. Likewise, you don't need to be severely ill to decide assisted living is the better option. Some seniors struggle with the right choice, especially when it feels like a close call. Some questions to ask yourself include:

- Would my health be at risk if I had to spend a few days alone in my home? If the answer is yes, you may need assisted living.
- Am I lonely but otherwise healthy? If yes, then independent living with its increased sense of community could be the best option.
- Am I relying more on my children or spouse to run errands or address regular needs? If so, assisted living could meet these needs.
- Do I have a serious medical condition? Assisted living can help if you have a serious diagnosis, particularly if that diagnosis is likely to get worse.
- Has my doctor expressed concern about me continuing to live alone? If so, consider assisted living.
- How do I feel being alone in my home? If you are anxious, this might mean you need assisted living. If you feel confident in your ability to care for yourself, but are bored or lonely, independent living could be the superior option.
- Have I let any daily activities, such as cooking, cleaning or bathing, fall by the wayside? Do I worry that these basic activities could be dangerous because of falling or another

"This desire to stay at home can often lead to unhealthy and isolated living conditions."

concern? If so, assisted living can offer some help and peace of mind.

BENEFITS OF MOVING TO SENIOR LIVING

Moving to a senior community isn't always the first choice for older adults. After all, living at home for as long as possible is considered healthy aging by most Americans. Many seniors try to stay at home for as long as they can, even while fighting chronic medical conditions, loneliness and memory loss. This desire to stay at home can often lead to unhealthy and isolated living conditions, which isn't healthy aging at all.

There is often a much better way to make friends, try new things and stay healthy—a senior living community! Senior living communities offer many benefits, including a lifestyle that keeps wellness at the forefront. Plus, senior living communities are often less expensive than living at home. If you need more reasons to consider senior living, here are few benefits that you may not have thought about.

Engaging Days

Senior living communities offer more than just medical care and daily assistance. For many seniors, living in a community means engaging, exciting and busy days. Residents often take classes at local colleges or universities, travel to local places of interest and have opportunities to learn a new language. There are cooking classes, gardening groups and ways to get into community leadership to make positive changes around you. Residents can participate in yoga classes and birding clubs, and they can volunteer at local organizations. Living in a senior living community means there is always something to do or somewhere to go, if you choose to do so.

Friendly Neighbors

Isolation can take a toll on seniors living alone at home. Research has shown that loneliness can lead to depression and even speed up the progression of dementia. In fact, perceived loneliness has been linked to cognitive decline. Fortunately, a senior living community is never lonely. With friendly faces and neighbors just steps down the hall, residents have a chance to actively build a support system of peers.

Lasting friendships and relationships with peers can decrease feelings of loneliness and depression, and friends can lead you to try something new. Healthy socialization gets residents out of their apartments and into meaningful conversations within their senior community, thus fostering feelings of connection and support.

Fewer Responsibilities

Finally, senior living community residents get the benefit of fewer household responsibilities. Without worrying about shoveling the sidewalk, mowing the yard, deep cleaning the home or doing the laundry, residents are able to focus on pursuing a life full of things they love. Senior living communities feature housekeeping, laundry, dining and maintenance services, all geared toward freeing up time for residents to pursue hobbies and other leisure.

Senior living communities are the best choice for healthy aging not only because of the access to medical assistance, but also because of the opportunities for engagement and socialization, and the ways they promote an active lifestyle focused on wellness.

Notes

Notes

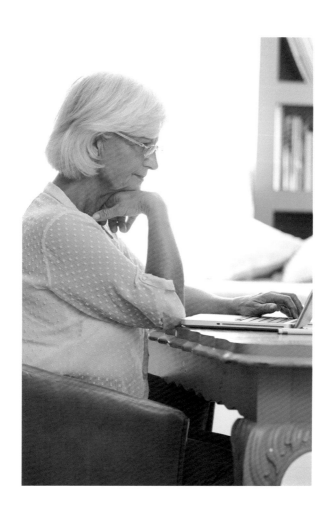

2 | *Beginning Your Search*

As challenging as it might be to make the initial decision to move to a senior living community, more difficult decisions loom, including determining the level of care you might need and finding the best community for you. Searching for the right community may take some time, but the effort is well worth it.

DO THE RESEARCH

Depending on where you live, you may be able to choose from dozens of senior living communities (or more). This range of options can seem daunting on the surface, but if you do your homework, you can find a community that meets all of your needs.

"Nothing can beat going to check out a community in person."

Where to Start

A simple Google search is an excellent way to begin searching for the right community. Most websites will provide basic information: location, amenities, care options and entertainment details, such as activities or nearby attractions. In addition to the community's website, read online reviews to get a sense of the quality of care and staff.

Although print brochures, virtual tours and online marketing materials all help narrow the search, nothing can beat checking out a community in person. You should go on a scheduled tour with a community representative who can answer all of your questions, but also pop in at other times, perhaps during a group activity or at mealtimes, so that you can see the interaction between staff and residents firsthand. Don't forget to ask one or two relatives to join on the visit—you can benefit from hearing their impressions. If you are serious about a senior living community but a little unsure about a particular facility, see if you can book a temporary stay; this can go a long way toward helping you make up your mind.

UNDERSTAND THE AVAILABLE OPTIONS IN SENIOR LIVING

If you have a special medical condition, you must determine if the community can provide the support required. Some specific considerations are outlined below.

Disability, Special Needs or Unique Medical Care

If a physical disability is present, it's important to choose a community that meets accessibility standards for both universal design and the Americans with Disabilities Act. These are some features that indicate a community's compliance:

Elevators

- Doorways and hallways that are wide enough to accommodate walkers and wheelchairs
- Easy-to-reach cupboards and shelves
- Bathrooms with grab bars and shower chairs
- Wheelchair-accessible apartments and showers
- Emergency call systems so you can call for assistance if needed

- Help for the visually impaired (find out if staff are trained to meet the needs of residents with low vision or complete vision loss)

Assisted Living

If you need help with any of the activities of daily living (eating, bathing, dressing, toileting, transferring/walking and continence), it's vital to find a community that provides the right amount of personal assistance and medical care. To find out if the residence will meet the your needs, ask the following questions:

- Does the community provide medication management?
- Does a licensed nurse complete a comprehensive individualized assessment for each resident? If so, how often are the assessments reviewed?
- How many nurses are on staff? Are they on site or accessible 24 hours a day?
- Does the community have visiting physicians? Home health services? On-site therapy/rehab services?

DETERMINE FINANCES

If finances are keeping you awake at night as

you try to figure out how to pay for senior living, you are not alone. Questions about the cost and affordability of senior living are usually among the first asked by seniors and their loved ones.

Senior living costs vary greatly across the country, which is why it's important to compare costs in your local market.

Important factors to consider when calculating the costs of senior living include which services and amenities you need, what is included in a particular senior living community's monthly rate and how much it would cost to arrange similar in-home services.

Calculating Your Current Costs

Calculating current and future living expenses is a great way to begin finding out how to pay for senior living. You can compare your current living expenses to different types of senior living and identify any services or amenities that are not currently necessary but will be needed in the future.

Many senior living options package living expenses such as housing, meals, entertainment, utilities, transportation and housekeeping together into a flat monthly fee. In other words, it's unnecessary to pay additional monthly

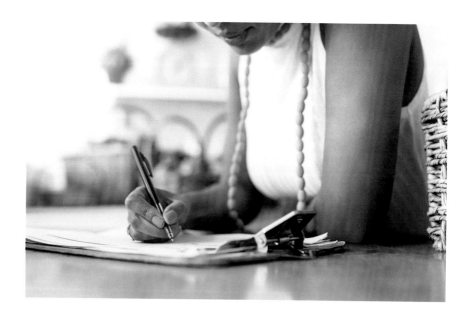

expenses for services such as groceries or a vehicle registration—unless you choose to purchase those things on your own. Independent senior living provides home health services in most communities, but does not offer its own 24-hour staff.

Use our interactive online price calculator at arborcompany.com/cost-calculator to add up the amount you pay for each of these expenses per month: mortgage or rent, utilities, home or renter's insurance, property tax, groceries, entertainment, lawn care and cleaning, maintenance or repairs, transportation and vehicle costs, home health services and other various costs, such as long-term care insurance or homeowner's association fees.

Once current living expenses are calculated down to the last cent, you can gauge the amount of additional monthly resources (if any) that should be added to the budget to pay for senior living.

Calculating Costs of Independent Senior Living

Independent senior living is often the most affordable senior living option. Residents typically don't require ongoing access to medical staff, assistance with everyday activities or help with medication management, so those services aren't included in monthly fees.

Independent senior living costs include shared or private apartments, meals, laundry and housekeeping, social activities, wellness activities and transportation services. All of the basic living expenses will be included in monthly rates. If you need home health services, such as medication management, these will not be included in the monthly rates.

Calculating Costs of Assisted Living

Assisted living is generally more expensive than independent senior living because costs include 24-hour supervision, access to medical staff, licensed on-site nurses and medication management services.

Residents might need help with normal daily activities such as bathing, dressing or eating. An assessment will be performed before you draft a personalized plan to meet your particular needs. The amount of help you need with activities of daily living (ADLs) will determine the best senior care option for you, and ultimately, your total monthly costs.

In addition to personal care, assisted living costs include shared or private apartments, meals, laundry and housekeeping, social programs, wellness programs and transportation services.

Adding It All Up

Your first step in calculating senior living costs should be to add up current expenses, including the costs of current or future in-home care needs. Then, as you calculate the costs of various types of senior living, you can compare those to your current costs and identify any new expenses that will be incurred.

Additional financial resources are available for seniors and families assessing how they will

"The amount of help you need with activities of daily living will determine the best senior care option for you."

———

pay for senior living. Four resources The Arbor Company recommends are:

- **ElderLifeFinancial.com:** ElderLife offers flexible line-of-credit programs that are ideal for those who need supplemental funding for senior living while they wait for other benefits to begin or are in the process of selling a home. These simple, convenient financing options are available to both residents and families.
- **LifeCareFunding.com:** Life Care Funding assists residents in liquidating life insurance policies through a Life Settlement program, which can assist in helping cover the costs of senior living when other assets such as a home or stocks are difficult to sell or are underperforming.
- **Tax deductibility benefit:** Present law provides that an individual can deduct from taxable income certain medical expenses associated

with living in nursing facilities, personal care homes and assisted living communities for the purpose of receiving medical care. This deduction may be applicable for adult children or certain other relatives who are paying a portion or all of a resident's costs associated with senior living. Consultation with a tax professional is strongly advised before making financial decisions.

- **Veterans Assistance Program:** Benefits are available for U.S. veterans or the surviving spouses of veterans. If you are eligible, you could receive a federal pension of approximately $2,000 per month to help pay for personal care such as assisted living. For more information, contact your local Department of Veteran Affairs.

Finally, remember that senior living costs vary greatly across the country, so it's important to diligently review costs in your specific region to get a true picture when calculating different types of senior living costs.

TOURING COMMUNITIES

All of your phone calls, emails, brochure reading and online research will help you inch

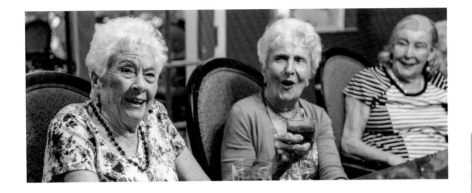

closer to a decision, but you won't truly get a feel for a senior living community without a tour. Here are some tips on what to look for and questions to ask during your visit to a potential new home.

Preparing for Your First Community Tour

When touring a potential community, several general things can be evaluated by simply looking around and asking the right questions. By beginning the tour with some idea of what you should be asking and looking for, you can ensure maximum comfort at the community you may soon call home.

Staff

For most, being surrounded by staff members who are kind, sociable and caring

"Observe how you are greeted by the receptionist and take note of how staff members engage with residents."

will beat living in a swanky environment any day. Right from the start, observe how you are greeted by the receptionist and take note of how staff members engage with residents. Do they come across as curt, cold or dismissive? Are they friendly, nurturing and patient? Also, be sure to ask about the staff-to-resident ratio—even the most caring workers may have little time for social interaction if they are constantly running in all directions to meet the needs of more residents than they can handle.

Leadership

Typically, it's a good sign if the community leadership staff—managers and directors—return phone calls promptly and courteously and answer all of your questions. Ask to meet the executive director and the resident care director on your tour. Take note of the way they greet you and whether or not they reach out to residents who cross their path.

Current Residents and Families

Dropping in several times should give you a general idea of a community's social atmosphere. Are residents out and about, talking and laughing with each other, or are you left with the impression that people generally keep to themselves or sit around all day? If you feel comfortable, strike up a conversation with a resident or two for their insight on the community. Because mealtime is a great opportunity for candid conversation, you might ask to join some residents at their table for lunch or dinner.

Keep in mind that as people give their opinions, they are bound to talk about what they find wrong with the community. These complaints shouldn't necessarily be dealbreakers—people will naturally like some parts of their home and dislike other parts. It will be your responsibility to weigh the good against the critical comments to form an overall impression of the community.

Amenities

In addition to housekeeping and laundry services, assisted living communities typically offer everything from wellness centers and gyms to chapels, hair salons and concierge services. They also usually provide plenty of common spaces, such as living rooms, libraries, clubhouses and business and internet centers.

Surroundings and Environment
There is no standard type of senior living community. Each one varies by design, ambience and atmosphere, ranging from high-rise apartments in the middle of a bustling downtown to campus communities surrounded by trees and greenery. As you begin a tour of any community, ask yourself if the setting appeals to you. If being outdoors is important, make sure there are plenty of gardens and patios, as well as places to sit in the sun, stroll around or even do some gardening.
When you go inside, what is your general impression of the building itself? Do you find the decor attractive and homey, or does it have an institutional feel? Listen carefully during your visit; are noise levels tolerable?

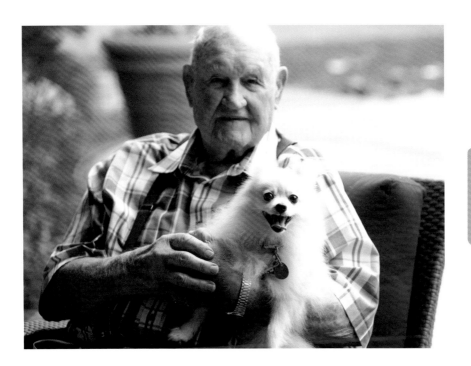

You may come across some communities that almost resemble vacation resorts. Keep in mind that the fanciest places are not necessarily the best communities. Most importantly, the building should be clean, fresh smelling and in good repair. Also, check for good natural and artificial lighting. Sunlight does wonders for the mind and body!

Although you should thoroughly appraise the dining hall, living rooms and other common areas, pay particular attention to the model apartment you are shown. This brief checklist will help you evaluate the space for comfortable living:

- Can you imagine your furniture in it?
- Do suites come with a kitchenette or at least a microwave and a mini fridge?
- Do you like the decor?

Activities and Entertainment

No senior living community will make residents participate in an activity if they don't want to, but it's important to recognize that getting involved is often the quickest way to feel at home. With that in mind, look at the community's event calendar to see if the scheduled activities are appealing. It's usually a good sign if the community offers a diverse range of activities, including ones geared to small-interest groups—think bird watching, book clubs or knitting groups—as well as larger, more inclusive events, such as garden parties or holiday celebrations. Also, find out if there are scheduled outings for trips to museums and the like.

On the tour, you may be able to speak to the activity director in order to find out if the preferences of residents are considered when developing the calendar. The best communities interview new residents and families to learn about what they like to do, as well as what they formerly enjoyed doing. These interviews are used to build community activity calendars so everyone can find some activities of interest.

Questions to Ask Staff and Administration

Understandably, you will have many questions during your tour—don't be afraid to ask. After all, the answers you receive will go a long way in helping you toward your decision. Keep some of these topics in mind as you learn more about a senior living community you are touring.

Food and Nutrition

Large senior living communities typically hire chefs and dietitians to ensure that meals are delicious, as well as nutritious. If possible, find out firsthand the quality of the food by sampling a meal. Look at a monthly or weekly menu in order to see which meal options are typically offered. Determine if residents ever help with menu planning and if there are any à la carte options. If you have a special diet, make sure that the kitchen can accommodate such requests.

Here are a few more questions to ask:

- When are mealtimes? Is there any flexibility around these times?
- What if a resident doesn't like items on the menu? Are there other options beyond something simple like chicken fingers?
- Are seats assigned in the dining room, or is it open/free seating?
- Can meals be eaten in private rooms or other locations (for example, in a café)?
- Are snacks available?

Freedom to Decorate and Rearrange

For many people transitioning to senior living, the prerogative to decorate and personalize their own living quarters is high on their list of priorities. If this is important to you, before any contract is signed, make sure you can bring your own belongings. This shouldn't be a problem with most, if not all, assisted living communities.

Visitation

Before you make a final decision on a particular community, establish that friends and family can visit whenever they like (within reason) and join you for a meal in the dining room if desired. It's a bonus if the community offers a separate dining room that you can book for special occasions such as birthdays or other family get-togethers. It's also a plus if the community allows the convenience and space for a grandchild or other visitor to spend the night in your apartment from time to time.

Options for Pets

If bringing the family tabby or hound is a must, make a point to inquire about pet policies. Some communities won't allow pets at all, and some that do have restrictions on the number or size of pets. If a community is pet-friendly, find out if grooming and dog walking services are available, as well as a pet coordinator who can help residents provide pet care if necessary. Take note that some "no pet" communities have a resident dog or cat. Some may even have a pet therapy program that allows seniors to interact on a regular basis with a therapy pet (usually a dog).

Transportation

If you still drive, confirm that the senior living community has a parking area for residents. If driving is no longer an option, life will be easier and more enjoyable if the community provides scheduled transportation to doctor or hairdressing appointments, as well as for shopping or other activities.

On-Site Rehabilitation

For residents with recurring injuries or the aches and pains of arthritis, on-site therapeutic options, such as massage, physical therapy or occupational therapy, can be convenient for rehabilitation. Also investigate whether the community offers group exercise programs that work to increase flexibility, balance and strength, such as tai chi, yoga or Pilates—including seated versions for those with mobility concerns.

Paying Attention to the Small Things

The primary features and amenities of a senior living community should be obvious during a tour. However, looking beyond the obvious—

and paying attention to the smaller details—is just as important in determining whether a community is right for your family. You can make a deeper assessment during a tour with these few tips:

- Request details about the specific accommodations you can expect. Ask if the unit you see on tour is similar to the one you would have.
- Seek insight from friends or family members who may think of needs you might not have considered. A second (or third) opinion is invaluable in making this decision about the next chapter of your life.
- Trust your instincts. Even if a place seems perfect on paper, listen to your gut if something tells you it's not right.

Narrowing Down Your List

If you tour multiple senior communities, be prepared for information overload. Understandably, you might struggle to remember what you liked and disliked about each community, or which location featured the best amenities. The Arbor Company offers a free, downloadable checklist (arborcompany.com/

checklist) that can help you compare features among multiple communities in one convenient check-the-box chart. Use the checklist to organize your opinions of the communities you toured and to help narrow down your list.

Once you have settled on a few top choices, returning for a second tour—or simply revisiting a community at a different time of day—can give you additional information as you work toward a decision. On your second visit, pay particular mind to the attentiveness of staff, the mood of residents, the cleanliness of the communities and other details you may have not noticed during the first tour. If you had gut feelings on your first visit, positive or negative, use the second to confirm those feelings or determine that you were mistaken.

A FINAL DECISION

Think carefully about the type of lifestyle that will truly make your senior years more enjoyable and stress-free. For instance, if your priorities are meeting people, socializing and entertainment, a large assisted living community in a busy metropolis might be a great fit. Alternatively, if mobility is a big concern, finding a place with on-site service providers—such as a hair salon or visiting physicians—might be top of mind in the overall evaluation.

Although one community may not fulfill all of your desires, at the very least you should create a short list of must-haves versus nice-to-haves— and never look for housing based on cost alone. Sometimes, a slightly higher price tag is worth the comfortable, carefree lifestyle that will allow for healthy and active senior years.

Whatever your priorities happen to be, the senior living community you choose can have a huge impact on your happiness, contentment and even health for years to come.

Notes

Notes

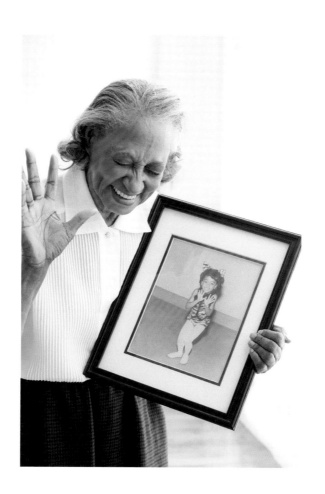

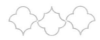

3 | *Making the Move*

Afterdeciding to move into senior living and choosing a community, the move itself might seem like the easy part of the journey. However, moving is never easy—you may experience powerful emotions leaving a home you lived in for decades. Take time with your move, and recognize it as a major step of the journey.

TIME TO DOWNSIZE

Your new senior living space or apartment might be smaller than the size of the home where you currently reside. If that is the case, you may need to downsize a bit. However, downsizing does not have to be something fear-inducing. In fact, it can be liberating! Streamlining your home before packing things into boxes can feel good. (There are companies that will help with downsizing and moving, if you prefer that route.)

In order to stay organized and make the most of your downsizing, consider these tips:

- Work room by room, drawer by drawer. Resist the urge to start a new project or move on to another room before completing the one you're currently working on.
- Designate categories for every item: keep, donate, give to someone special, sell, throw away.
- Take photos of favorite things that you won't keep; these photographs can be made into an album that you will cherish for years to come.
- Remember that things are things; they are not memories. You can have memories forever, even if you don't have the things.
- If you aren't quite sure what to do with a certain item, put it down and sleep on your decision. Anyone can make poor decisions when feeling tired or overwhelmed.
- Resist the urge to keep items in a rented storage area. You will not want to repeat this

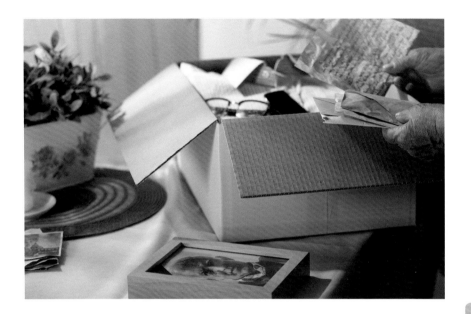

downsizing process in a few years with the items you shuffled out to your storage unit. Bite the bullet and make the decisions now.

- Consider keeping holiday decorations on a reduced scale. Most senior communities encourage residents to make their apartments feel like home, and putting up a festive wreath or other items can certainly help. Just remember that you will be decorating a smaller space, so it is best to avoid toting along the seven-foot Christmas tree and opt for a small tree instead.

Although your personal style and situation may dictate the items that you decide to bring

"Bring your favorite and most comfortable pieces—but consider every season."

———

to the new apartment, there are a few universal categories to consider:

Clothing

You may be moving into a home with a smaller closet than you currently have. Here are a few tips for deciding what clothing to bring:

- Take time to evaluate each piece. If it doesn't fit or hasn't been worn for a year or longer, don't bring it.
- If you are moving to a senior community with a four-season climate, don't forget to pack items for each season.
- Bring your favorite and most comfortable pieces—but consider every season.
- Don't forget to bring loungewear, pajamas and a cozy robe.
- Go easy on shoes. It is best to bring a few pairs of comfortable shoes for daily wear, such as tennis shoes.

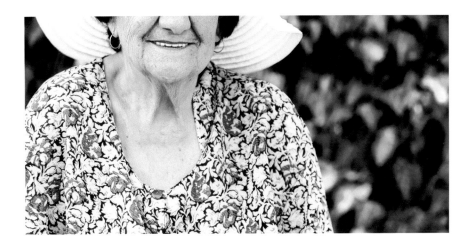

- If there is a laundry service at the community, determine if you need to label clothing according to any policy. Take care of this before the move so that you won't have to worry about it on your first laundry day.
- If you will be doing your own laundry, remember to bring a laundry basket or hamper, along with your favorite detergent and supplies.

Furniture

At most senior living apartments, residents are given an empty space ready to be filled with their own furniture. Consider a few of these ideas when loading up furniture:

- Ask about items provided by the facility and

which larger pieces you may bring in.

- Measure the new apartment, and keep a floor plan handy while making decisions. Nothing is more frustrating than realizing on moving day that the king-sized bed cannot fit into the new bedroom.
- Consider selling some large items and investing in smaller, more apartment-friendly furniture. For example, a small loveseat and chair might be a much better fit for the new living room than a large, bulky sectional from home.
- If you have a "must come" piece, be ready for the possibility that you may have to sacrifice something else. If a beloved piano is a priority, you might have to forgo bringing a lounge chair; there simply may not be enough space.
- Consider pieces that serve more than one function. A coffee table with drawers, for example, does double duty to enhance your storage.
- Speaking of storage, a well-placed shelving or drawer unit in the bathroom can do wonders. Drawers in the bathroom can provide some extra space or eliminate the need for a linen closet.

Decor

Personal style doesn't need to diminish when moving into a senior living community! Consider these tips when packing decor:

- Planning to hang art or photos? Keep your floor plan and measurements handy so you'll know how much you can bring on move-in day.
- Resist the urge to pack large pieces of art or cabinetry. In addition to furniture, these extras can make the new home seem cramped and can even become a mobility or tripping hazard.
- Speaking of tripping hazards, be wary of rugs. Unsecured rugs can cause residents to slip and trip. If you do bring rugs, make sure they are skid-proof and secured.
- Be realistic when packing up infrequently used items. For example, the huge Thanksgiving serving platters will only take up cabinet space in a new home.

Personal Items

Finally, bring along those extra special items that you love, using these tips for consideration:

- Photos are great, and some should be taken

along. However, there may not be room to hang all of the photos that fit in the old home. Pick out favorites, and slide the others into albums that you can easily store on a bookshelf.

- Bring along your must-have items only if you know something similar is not already available. For example, consider leaving behind the coffee pot if coffee is served every morning right down the hall.

- Don't forget to bring along a smartphone, tablet or computer to stay connected. However, if you can pare down electronics because there is a computer lab on campus, consider doing so.

- Don't forget to bring medical necessities, including medical information, prescriptions (as necessary), doctor information and emergency contact information. Most of these items will be collected ahead of time, but having them just in case is wise.

What Not to Pack

As you finalize the packing list, remember that moving into a senior living community means letting go of certain possessions. Here are a few things to consider leaving behind:

- **Cleaning supplies:** Amenities at senior living communities include regular housekeeping services. Say "so long" to deep cleaning, and leave your cleaning supplies behind. Consider bringing light supplies, such as bleach wipes or a dust cloth.
- **Oversized furniture:** Remember to keep floor plan measurements handy as you consider which furniture to bring to your new living space. Slimmed-down, apartment-friendly choices will keep the home feeling spacious and safe.
- **Your entire book, puzzle or other collection:** If you have a large collection of items (books, puzzles, figurines, games and so on), consider bringing only a few favorites. Large collections can make the new space feel cramped; bringing just a few favorites can give a nod to your personality and style without sacrificing the space.
- **Extravagant jewelry:** Jewelry can certainly be an important part of your personal story and style. However, for any large collection of pricey pieces, consider putting the majority of the items in a safety deposit box or other location outside of your new apartment.

THE MOVE-IN PROCESS

After putting down a deposit and selecting a residence, you will be ready to move in, but there are a few remaining steps. The move itself—arriving at the community and getting situated—requires some planning.

If you have planned ahead for the move into your new community, there will be time before move-in day to enjoy activities, meals or other welcoming opportunities. These events are the perfect way for you to ease into community living by meeting key staff members and new neighbors or friends. Accept these invitations and bring family members along for a familiar face and touchstone of support.

For assisted living, after the initial deposit has made things official, a representative from the community will come to your home to perform an assessment. This assessment gives the staff the opportunity to get to know you a bit better and assess needs, challenges and preferences. It is best for the community to have some of this baseline information before you move in so that the staff can be prepared to work with you beginning your first day at the community.

Depending on state regulations, the community may ask you to visit your physician prior to move in. The doctor will need to forward some state-mandated paperwork to the assisted living community. Don't worry—the community will provide you with that paperwork if it is necessary in your state.

With any type of senior living community, you will work with a representative from the community to complete some standard move-in paperwork. This paperwork typically consists of a standard rental agreement, along with other information that may ease the transition.

The move itself will be well-coordinated and scheduled by the team at the community. You will receive a time frame in which to arrive. You will most likely be greeted with a welcome basket in the new apartment, and a representative from the community will give you a walk-through tour of your new home. You will receive your apartment keys and any wearable technology that the assisted living community may provide, such as pendants to push in case of emergency.

It's possible to put in a work request to have maintenance staff members help hang a shelf or favorite photos in the days to come. Be sure to eat amid all of the excitement; a staff representative will stop by to escort you to the dining room.

Moving day is sure to be full of excitement and stress. Family can help ease your transition by simply being there to help with unpacking, coordinating movers, the contract signing or to simply join you for your first meal at your new home. A familiar presence can go a long way for calming nerves and reaffirming your decision to move.

SETTLING IN

There are other ways for you to make your new space feel like home when you move in. Bring a bit of personality to your new space by considering a few of these tips:

- **Hang photos first:** Although putting furniture in the best places is certainly important, hanging or displaying some favorite photos upon moving in can create a sense of welcome. Pictures will provide a reminder of home and give new neighbors and staff members something to talk about when they greet you in your new apartment.

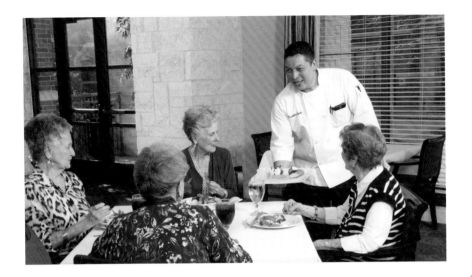

- **Enjoy a meal:** Head down to the dining room for a meal! Not only will you enjoy delicious food that you didn't have to prepare, but you will also be able to meet some new friends. It is always great to see smiling faces at dinner.
- **Add a welcome sign:** Something as simple as hanging a sign on the apartment door can do wonders for feeling at home. It can also be an indication that you are eager to meet new neighbors.
- **Dress your windows:** Most communities will allow residents to repaint the walls in their rooms—within reason—but this may be more work than you want to undertake. An easier alternative is choosing your own window treatments. This freedom to express

yourself can add some color and style to your new home.

- **Host friends:** Welcome friends—new and old—into your home as soon as possible after the move. You don't need to host something elaborate to feel genuine—simply brew a pot of coffee (or ask for a pot to be brought in) and put some cookies on a plate. Other residents will love meeting their new neighbor, and old friends will love checking out your new home. Don't be shy about showing off the new space!
- **Unpack and explore:** The new space will begin to feel like home when you associate it with relaxation and coziness. The best way to make a new home a safe haven is to get out and explore the new community. Take advantage of meals in the dining room, as well as group activities. You will meet new friends, explore new hallways and look forward to returning to your cozy home.

If you feel a bit disoriented after moving into your senior living community, don't worry. It is normal to feel overwhelmed for a few weeks or even months. Be honest with your family and with the staff about your feelings.

Notes

Notes

Notes

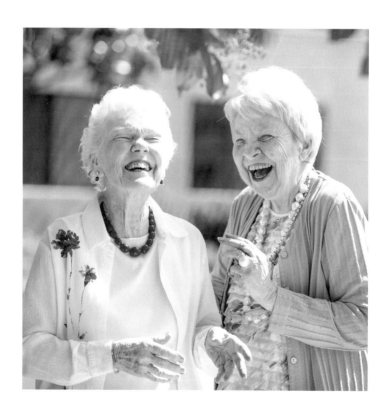

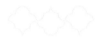

4 | *Conclusion*

The journey to senior living takes time, research, and plenty of patience. There may be tears and triumphs along the way, and hopefully, the end result will be a community where you or your loved one finds happiness, friendship and health.

The Arbor Company brings three decades of excellence and experience to independent living, assisted living and memory care. With more than three dozen communities in 10 states, we set the standard in senior living and are committed to our residents and their families. Take a tour today to learn more.

Even if you don't choose an Arbor community or do not live in an area where we operate, we hope you enjoyed this comprehensive guide and that you will subscribe to our blog (blog. arborcompany.com) to learn more about senior living. We also recommend using some of our tools at the end of this book.

Finally, if you have any questions about our senior living communities, don't hesitate to visit our online contact page (www.arborcompany. com/contact-us) or call us at 404-237-4026. We look forward to hearing from you!

FREQUENTLY ASKED QUESTIONS

Even after reading through our comprehensive guide, you may still have questions. This FAQ answers some of those questions. Again, contact us (www.arborcompany.com/contact-us) if we have not covered your question in this guide.

Assisted Living

Is assisted living different from a nursing home?
Yes. The Arbor Company's assisted living communities are residential living communities that provide supportive assistance and also coordinate care with other providers in each resident's home. As a community of caregivers, we are committed to engaging and enriching

the health and spirit of our residents. We honor individuality and develop deep connections with our residents, families and staff.

How do you know it's time for assisted living?
Change is difficult, but it's essential that you not wait for a crisis to dictate a move into assisted living. In fact, many families are surprised that assisted living actually makes their loved one more independent and wish they had moved sooner. Residents are offered the exact amount of support they need, without having to rely on family members or friends for various tasks.

By exploring your options now, you will have more time to make an informed decision and weigh your choices. This also ensures you choose the right community, instead of choosing a community solely based on availability. As you consider whether now is the time, take into account safety and quality of life. An assisted living community provides healthy meals and clinical oversight, but it also provides laughter, support and a true sense of community. It's a place where friendships are formed and life is lived to the fullest every day. And guess what? Someone else will clean up after your party!

Is the staff well-trained? How can I tell?

To get a sense of the type of care offered at a particular community, you should schedule a tour and come with questions such as:

- How does the assisted living community staff care for the resident's needs?
- How many registered nurses, licensed practical nurses and personal support workers are on staff? (Look for a community that has a licensed nurse on duty or on call at all times.)
- How many staff members work at any given time, including overnights?
- What is the staff members' training in such areas as safety, emergency care, first aid, mental health, residents' rights and medication administration?

Once you've taken a tour, drop in once or twice, perhaps during a mealtime or activity, to observe how staff interacts with residents.

Are there roommates?

Companion living options are available at most assisted living communities. Couples are also welcome!

Is anyone not eligible for assisted living?

Assisted living is not designed for adults needing 24-hour nursing services. Each state has regulations that mandate the level of care we can provide in our assisted living and memory care communities. Contact an Arbor care counselor for a personalized assessment to see if assisted living is right for you.

How can family members check on care?

Family members can relax knowing their loved ones are being cared for 24 hours a day. If an issue arises, we will notify the family and work together to resolve it. Rest assured that residents' family members can visit any time. Often, family members take residents home for visits, errands or any other number of reasons.

Is travel still possible?

Residents may travel as they wish, as long as it is cleared by their physician.

Independent Living

What is independent living?

Arbor Company's full-service independent living communities offer a maintenance-free lifestyle with numerous amenities and luxury

"These communities focus on providing a comfortable, independent lifestyle, but also offer peace of mind if a health issue arises."

---

services to fit your every want and need. These communities focus on providing a comfortable, independent lifestyle, but also offer peace of mind if a health issue arises. Our residents are surprised at the amount of independence they have. For example, you will still purchase toiletries such as soap, shampoo, tissue and toilet paper.

Will I be the youngest/oldest person in the community?

Each Arbor community is home to residents of varying ages, but one thing is for sure: Age is nothing but a number. You won't notice if you are the youngest or oldest person in the community; most likely, you will be too busy to ask. Communities cater to a wide range of interests, with activities that stimulate residents physically, mentally and socially.

How independent is it, really?

At an independent senior living community, you have complete freedom with your time and living space. You can participate in social and recreational events—or not. You can come and go as you please. As for food, independent living communities often offer custom-designed meal packages, thus allowing residents to choose a specified number of meals per day.

Is driving an option?

Absolutely! Many residents still drive their own cars, so parking is available at most communities. For those who choose not to drive, most residences offer a private bus for local shopping and day trips.

Is it possible to travel?

There are no restrictions on travel whatsoever. In fact, travel is easier and more worry-free than ever thanks to the security of knowing that your home will be safe while you're gone.

Can I drink alcohol?

Yes! In most independent living communities, alcohol is permitted. Some faith-based communities may have an alcohol-free policy, so be sure to ask when touring community options.

Conclusion

Can I have overnight guests?

Yes! Your apartment is just that: yours. If you would like to entertain and invite friends and family for a visit, you are more than welcome to do so.

What's the difference between independent living and a 55+ community or senior apartments?

In an independent living community, residents live in accessible apartments and have access to a number of common areas, such as game rooms, libraries, business centers and more. These communities provide numerous social and recreational activities on- and off-site. Premium independent living areas often include:

- Delicious home-cooked meals
- Transportation
- Housekeeping and laundry
- Fitness facilities
- Beauty salons
- Concierge services

There is on-site security, a 24-hour emergency help call system, and often, a nurse on staff during weekday business hours.

Senior and 55+ community apartments are similar to independent living communities, but offer few organized social activities or care services. They do offer such amenities as fitness centers, tennis courts, pools and golf course access, and they typically have community gates and security patrol.

What happens in the case of an illness?
Many senior living options include on-site first aid and nursing care in case of emergencies. Other communities can provide nursing staff or personal companions for a fee. However, the medical services available in an independent living community are governed by state regulations, so it's important to ask questions up front about the type of assistance the community is legally able to provide.

Is there a benefit to independent living if assistance isn't needed?
At an independent living community, time isn't wasted on keeping up with housework and other daily chores, which means you can devote more of your energy to enjoying recreational activities, learning new skills and looking after your physical, emotional, social and spiritual well-being.

"Keep in mind that regardless of the type of unit, you can furnish and decorate it as you wish."

———

Can the environment and setting be personalized?
Independent living communities do not come in a single blueprint. You could live in a large high-rise apartment in a downtown neighborhood or in a smaller community with a small-town feel. Units vary in size from a studio to a full apartment. In some communities, residents live in condos, townhouses or small cottages. Also, keep in mind that regardless of the type of unit, you can furnish and decorate it as you wish. In fact, paint colors or carpeting are often customizable, just like with an apartment or home rental.

What happens when the care required doesn't allow for independent living?
In some cases, one can remain in an independent living community as long as the family or a home healthcare provider provides caregiving. Another option is to move to an

assisted living community. Many independent living and assisted living communities share the same campus, thus making the move easier.

Senior Living

How much does it cost?

Costs vary based on location, amenities and services, among other factors. Arbor Company communities accommodate a range of budgets.

Does Medicare cover the cost?

Medicare does not cover the rent and care costs of independent living, and its coverage of assisted living is limited to pharmacy, rehab and other services through Medicare Part B.

Is customization available for meal plans?

Yes. Our team works hard to customize meals to specific dietary requirements, including allergies.

Notes

Conclusion

Notes

ADDITIONAL RESOURCES

SENIOR LIVING OPTIONS QUIZ
Which type of senior living option is right for you?

Transitioning into senior living can be a difficult process without having the right information. One of the biggest questions is determining which level of care is right for you. The goal of this quiz is to answer that question and to help you take the next step with confidence.

1. How well are you able to move around?

☐ I can move around independently.
1 point

☐ I can move around with assistance from a cane, walker or wheelchair.
2 points

☐ I can move around but need occasional assistance from others.
2 points

☐ I can't move around without assistance due to physical limitations and/or confusion.
3 points

Point Total _____

2. If you use a wheelchair, can you transfer in and out by yourself?

☐ I am not in a wheelchair.
   1 point

☐ Yes.
   1 point

☐ No.
   2 points

Point Total _____

3. How often do you experience falls?

☐ I rarely fall.
   1 point

☐ I occasionally fall but can get up on my own.
   1 point

☐ I occasionally fall and need assistance getting up.
   2 points

☐ I often fall and can't get up.
   2 points

Point Total _____

4. How often do you experience falls? How much help do you need with transportation?

☐ I can independently drive and maintain a vehicle, or I am able to use public transportation on my own.
1 point

☐ I need help arranging transportation but am fine taking it on my own.
1 point

☐ I could use someone to help arrange transportation and come with me to appointments and to do shopping
2 points

☐ I require transportation to appointments and to go shopping due to physical restrictions or confusion.
3 points

Point Total _____

5. How much help do you need during meals?

☐ None.
1 point

☐ I need help getting to the dining room.
2 points

☐ I have a hard time using utensils.
2 points

☐ I rely on someone else during meals.
2 points

Point Total _____

6. How well are you able to dress and undress?

☐ I can independently dress and undress myself.
1 point

☐ I need assistance dressing and undressing myself.
2 points

Point Total _____

7. How well are you able to groom yourself and perform proper hygiene?

☐ I can independently bathe and groom myself.
1 point

☐ I can independently bathe and groom myself, but I occasionally need reminders.
2 points

☐ I can bathe and groom myself, but I need supervision.
2 points

☐ I need physical assistance bathing and grooming myself.
2 points

Point Total _____

8. How well are you able to use the restroom?

☐ I can independently use the toilet and maintain proper hygiene.
1 point

☐ I am incontinent but able to maintain hygiene with proper supplies.
1 point

☐ I need occasional assistance with problems related to incontinence.
2 points

☐ I am unable to manage incontinence and need physical assistance with bathroom use.
2 points

Point Total _____

9. How easily can you see a physician on your own?

☐ I can independently schedule and keep all appointments without assistance.
1 point

☐ I can schedule and keep all appointments but need assistance from others.
2 points

☐ I need appointments scheduled for me.
2 points

Point Total _____

10. What daily medical needs do you experience that require help from a skilled nurse or other healthcare professional?

☐ Oxygen **2 Points**
☐ Intravenous feeding/fluids **S**
☐ Injections/insulin therapy **2 Points**
☐ Physical therapy **2 Points**
☐ Catheter care **S**
☐ Other **S**
☐ None **1 point**

Number of S's_____   Point Total _____

11. How well are you able to manage your own medications?

☐ I can independently take all medications.
1 point

☐ I need occasional reminders to take medications.
1 point

☐ I need physical assistance in measuring correct doses or applying medication.
2 Points

☐ I need complete assistance.
2 Points

Point Total _____

12. How good is your memory?

☐ I am completely aware of surroundings, recognize and remember people, and know dates and times without reminders.
1 point

☐ I have difficulty remembering names, the date and/or time of day.
2 Points

☐ I have trouble remembering things that happened recently.
2 Points

☐ I do not recognize familiar people and am unable to recognize date, time and/or surroundings.
M

Number of M's_____   **Point Total** _____

13. How well do you handle your emotions?

☐ I can handle emotions without difficulty, cope with stress and get along well with others.
1 point

☐ I prefer to isolate myself from others.
2 Points

☐ I often experience periods of frustration, anxiety and/or agitation that need intervention.
2 Points

Point Total _____

14. If you can walk/get around independently, have you experienced any of the following?

☐ Being somewhere without knowing how you arrived.
M

☐ Taking longer than usual to return home from a walk or a drive.
2 Points

☐ Feeling like you needed to be someplace even though you were at home.
M

☐ Forgetting directions to familiar places, either inside or outside.
2 Points

Additional Resources

☐ I have not experienced any of these situations.
1 Point

Number of M's_____ **Point Total** _____

Results
(13-18 points) Independent Living

Independent living is for healthy, active seniors who require little or no support with activities of daily living (ADLs). Residents choose how active to be. For example, they may decide to cook all their own meals, enjoy meals in the community dining room with friends or plan their dining options somewhere in between. Independent living emphasizes that this is the time for seniors to enjoy life to the fullest, in any way they see fit.

(19-26 points) Assisted Living

The best assisted living delivers outstanding service, providing as much help as necessary for seniors to enjoy active, engaging lives. Communities offer varying levels of care based on a resident's needs with activities of daily living (ADLs) and medical requirements. Assisted living fills in the gaps that seniors might otherwise struggle with.

(Choosing Answer Marked M) Memory Care
Memory care communities offer many of the amenities (personalized attention, help with activities of daily living, medical care and more) of assisted living, but with a focus on care for residents with Alzheimer's disease or other dementias. Activities and routines are structured with the goal of maximizing the independence, engagement and livelihood of residents.

(Choosing Answer Marked S) Skilled Nursing
Skilled nursing offers a 24-hour level of care for patients with more particular medical needs that can be met only by someone with advanced training, such as a registered nurse (RN) or a licensed practical nurse (LPN). Other services may be provided by certified nursing assistants (CNAs). Skilled nursing may include administration of medicine and injections, physical and occupational therapy, catheter care or intravenous feeding.

Disclaimer: This quiz is just a general overview of which level of care may be right for you. Call your senior care counselor for a private consultation on which level is right for you.

COMPARE THE COST OF SENIOR LIVING TO STAYING AT HOME

Are you able to afford senior living? We've created this cost of senior living calculator to help you understand the costs of senior living versus the costs of aging in place. To estimate the cost of your options, simply fill in your current expenses and let us know the level of care you think is right for you.

Step 1: Current Costs

Calculate your current at-home expenses in this table.

At-Home Expenses	Monthly Costs
Mortgage or rent payment (e.g., $190)	
Total of utilities (e.g., $245)	
Home or renters insurance (e.g., $45)	
Property Tax (e.g., $225)	
Grocery and Food (e.g. $200)	
Entertainment, hobbies, and so on. (e.g., $200)	
Lawn care and cleaning services (e.g., $440)	

At-Home Expenses	Monthly Costs
Maintenance or repairs (e.g. $20)	
Transportation (vehicle insurance, registration, gas, maintenance, and repairs) (e.g. $200)	
Current or anticipated home healthcare/companion costs (The average national monthly cost is $3,360-$5,760.)	
Total Monthly At-Home Costs	

Step 3: Care Level

Choose the care type or living option you think is a fit.

Independent Living - $4,730*

Independent living is for healthy, active seniors who require little or no support with activities of daily living (ADLs). Residents choose how active they want to be. For example, they may decide to cook all their meals, enjoy meals in the community dining room with friends or plan their dining options somewhere in between. Independent living emphasizes that this is the time for seniors to enjoy life to the fullest, in any way they see fit.

Additional Resources

Assisted Living - $4,968*

The best assisted living delivers outstanding service to residents, providing as much help as necessary for seniors to enjoy active, engaging lives. Communities offer varying levels of care based on a resident's needs with activities of daily living (ADLs) and medical requirements. Assisted living fills in the gaps that seniors might otherwise struggle with.

Memory Care - $6,118*

Memory care communities offer many of the amenities (personalized attention, help with activities of daily living, medical care and more) of assisted living, but with a focus on care for residents with Alzheimer's disease or other dementias. Activities and routines are structured with the goal of maximizing the independence, engagement and livelihood of residents.

Skilled Nursing - $6,943*

Skilled nursing offers a 24-hour level of care for patients with more particular medical needs that can be met only by someone with advanced training, such as a registered nurse (RN) or a licensed practical nurse (LPN).

Other services may be provided by certified nursing assistants (CNAs). Skilled nursing may include administration of medicine and injections, physical and occupational therapy, catheter care or intravenous feeding.

This information is based on national data and does not reflect regional price variations.

Step 4: Compare Costs

Compare your monthly costs of living at home to the national average monthly cost of the care level that may be right for you.

Total Monthly At-Home Costs	National Average Monthly Cost of Care

**Keep in mind, supplemental resources may cover 50-100 percent of your monthly fees in a senior community. A veteran's pension or life insurance plan may apply and long-term care policies can contribute $90-120 per day of care costs, or roughly $3,660 per month on average.*

SENIOR LIVING EVALUATION CHECKLIST

	Community Name			
First Impressions				
The exterior of the building is well maintained.				
The community feels like home.				
I was welcomed in a warm and gracious manner.				
Communication				
All of my requests are responded to within 24 hours.				
I feel staff communication is clear and delivered in a timely manner.				
The community encourages honest, open and caring feedback.				
My feedback is valued through a satisfaction survey process.				

	Community Name			
Community Culture				
The privacy and dignity of seniors is of great importance.				
All staff work as a team and treat each other with respect.				
The community has reputable affiliations and partnerships.				
People				
All staff are warm, caring and competent.				
There is a consistent execution of effort from all staff.				
Ongoing staff training is provided.				
The community places importance on staff retention.				

Additional Resources

Community Name			
Deep Connections			
An effort is made to personally know each resident.			
Staff engage in meaningful interactions with residents and family.			
An engagement program is in place, offering individualized options.			
Special events are planned to honor milestones for each resident.			
Resident Care			
The community offers personalized care, recognizing preferences.			
Care is delivered "like a friend."			
Ongoing assessments are conducted and reviewed with family.			
Staff are trained as Dementia Care Specialists.			

	Community Name			
Resident Care (continued)				
On-site therapy and rehabilitation is available.				
Specialized care programs such as diabetic management are offered.				
Licensed nurses are on staff.				
Accountability and Financial Solutions				
The management company has been in business for over 25 years.				
The community conducts personal affordability assessments.				
Financial assessments are available (VA assistance, Elderlife, and so on.)				
The community places importance on staff retention.				

We understand that finding the right senior living community for your loved one is extremely important. That's why we encourage you to compare us to our competition.

Additional Resources